# It Started with a Green Dress:

Overcoming Sexual Stigma

DESTINY MARIA

IT STARTED WITH A GREEN DRESS
*Copyright © 2020 by Destiny Maria*

*ISBN-13:* 978-0-578-65483-6

*To those who fear disclosure and suffer in silence.*

# TABLE OF CONTENTS

# DISCLAIMER

*The following is a portrayal of my individual journey. There were many hardships I faced prior to my diagnosis. Difficult life circumstances and lack of resources fueled my depression. In no way does it reflect the quality of life for someone living with a positive status. Not everyone experiences such intense symptoms. Please keep this in mind when reading the emotion exacerbated in this book.*

# PREFACE

The gift that keeps on giving; that's right. This book is about exactly what you think it is. But I'll tell you what it isn't. It isn't a lecture. And it isn't a recap of what we've all learned about STDs/ STIs and prevention. Yes, I'm talking about sexually transmitted diseases and infections. Because guess what? The slideshows and graphic images in our textbooks weren't the whole truth.

For as long as I knew, only dirty or promiscuous people contracted STDs. And if you have one, you're going to give it to everyone you sleep with! The goal seems to remain "clean" while avoiding unplanned pregnancy. Horrific images of puss-filled blisters and sores or indescribable objects on genitalia left my stomach in knots. Pictures on the internet only added to the fear of what could happen "down there."

If I ever caught something like that I would die. Then there's the common assumption you'd have to be sleeping with multiple partners, too many to count, in order to catch a disease. We all know the woman at work who sleeps with everyone at the office. Or the man who will give it to just about anything that walks. They must have *something*. You may be saying to yourself, not me. I know the person I'm sleeping with, I trust them. I don't sleep around. My partner told me they don't have anything so they must be good to go. My favorite are those who believe condom use will protect you 100% from contracting any wart, bump, or unwanted excess discharge.

Well, I'm here to tell you the many unpleasant truths about sex. First and foremost, CONDOMS DO NOT FULLY PROTECT YOU AGAINST STDs/STIs. This includes the incurables. But what if I'm a virgin? I couldn't possibly be at risk.

Second false assumption would be: It doesn't matter if you've had zero, one, two, or a thousand partners. You are still at risk of contracting an STD. You can contract an STI without sex! This book is about one in particular. I am the one of the many faces of the gift that keeps on giving. When I contracted this "gift" everything I had ever known became a lie. It isn't a gift and shouldn't be referred to as one. To help cope, a friend of mine recommended I write a book to share my story with the world.

In an attempt to end our wide spread miseducation on a large portion of the population - those of us living with a positive status. This book is for you. And for those who test negative, prepare to open your minds and break through the barriers that keep the stigma alive. As we buy into the idea of what someone should look or act like in order to have an STD we are promoting non-disclosure; sex without informative consent. This lessens the likelihood of STD positives informing their partners. And YOU could be one of them. So, the next time you make a joke about sexually transmitted diseases, you could be hurting someone close to you or highly offending the person beside you.

*This is my story. My experience. Our reality. And it all started with a green dress.*

# Chapter 1

# DEVASTATION

⟶

"Trust me this is not as bad as it seems."
I stare at the text message as his words linger in my mind. I lay there.

*Lifeless.*

As if the world stopped for a moment.

*Damaged.*

I no longer felt like an object of desire. The blister throbbed as I tried not to look. I slept. Hours passed and I wished to awake from my reality. But it doesn't end and it won't. He said he'll pay my medical expenses. As if that were enough for a lifelong disease.

*Betrayal.*

He asks what he can do to make it better. The truth is; nothing. There is nothing he can do to heal the emotional pain.

"How could you do this to me?" My voice trembled.

They say the first outbreak is the worst. It gets better in time. He took my youth. The beauty that came with being young and free vanished in an instant. I would never be the same.

Who will want me now?

*Insecure.*

My confidence has been stripped from me. I hated myself once more. Was this some sort of cruel punishment? I was given a printout of my diagnosis along with home care instructions. The virus comes with a vicious stigma. A stigma I can't escape. I'm labeled promiscuous. Someone you don't want to have sex with.

You fear contraction.

I fear transmission.

Society says I should be ashamed of myself for my decisions. But I'm no different from most. He says I have my whole life ahead of me; it doesn't stop me from living. I was only twenty-two years old. He didn't understand. Maybe he's forgotten what it's like. The beginning can be painfully unpredictable. I close my eyes praying that when they open, I am free.

"This isn't real," I tell myself.

What will my family think? The thought of a parents' nightmare come true. I decided to keep my secret.

Don't ask, don't tell.

I never had much emotional support from my family. Miscommunication was the greatest distance between us. Keeping it from them ate me up inside. My eyes water, I don't recognize myself as I'm unable to upkeep my usual appearance. I cried nonstop for days. My stomach ached from barely eating. I avoided using the restroom as the stinging was a constant reminder of my mistake. It burned. One sore caused excruciating pain. Something so small, hardly noticeable became impossible to ignore. I trusted him to be honest with me. But everyone has their own definition of honesty.

Each morning is different. Some days begin with depression; then other days in anger and resentment. Frustrated with myself and his replies, "Destiny I am truly sorry for everything. Please let me know how I can help make this less painful," his text message read.

How am I supposed to receive help from the person who caused me harm?

I could feel my heart breaking. Shattering into pieces like glass. My eyes swell with tears running down my cheeks. I'm struggling to come to terms with the new me. I missed work several times in the past 2 weeks. I need time to adjust. But life doesn't stop for anyone. It was 4:30 pm and I had been in bed since our last phone call. It was the conversation that changed my entire life.

His truth finally revealed.

Things don't always happen the way we expect them to. I didn't expect him to say what he did.

I'm *devastated.*

Left to pull myself together as he'd asked me to. I was drowning. I'm not sure what I wanted him to say. Perhaps, I needed to hear something that would make me feel "normal" again. I was routinely tested prior and wanted to live my life as freely as possible. I guess he did too.

*Guilt.*
*Shame.*

*Embarrassment.*

My friends say I'll get through this. Without them, I'd be lost with nowhere to run and nowhere to hide. You see, I've been hurt and left with disappointment many times in my life. But this was an unfamiliar pain. One I hadn't experienced before. This was a different kind of heartache.

It wasn't a romantic relationship. It was sex. No strings attached. Casual sex is considerably more acceptable in today's society. Others choose not to engage in it for their own reasoning. I'm not trying to convince anyone they shouldn't hook up. What I am doing is sharing my personal experience of what isn't discussed when it comes to sex.

He misled me.

I thought I knew him. Not entirely, but at least to have an understanding as to what kind of a person he was. I didn't. Because when you're casually hooking up with someone, you don't really know the person you're sleeping with. We go to bed with their persona. He hid behind a mask. The mask we all carry to hide who or what we are inside. I once read a theory that says you have three faces. The first face, you show to the rest of the world. The second, you show to loved ones, your family. The third face, you show no one. It's the truest reflection of who you are. I understand it now more than ever.

My thoughts race with signs I should've seen coming. Things he said, things he did. I somehow managed to force myself out of bed. I could feel the itch as I limped to the restroom. I've made some poor decisions in the past. I'm sure this wasn't the last of it. I rinse my hands in the sink carefully glancing at my skin. The paranoia of spreading it to other parts of my body began to sink in. Would I wake up one morning covered in sores? I should've protected myself. But I wasn't accepting that this unfortunate circumstance had nothing to do with me and everything to do with him. Growing up, I was taught prevention, not to share cups or kiss relatives on the lips. Condoms were the ideal way to promote sexual health and help prevent pregnancy. The worst outcome was to catch an incurable disease. Fear-based thinking is incredibly powerful.

We tend to forget we're not invincible. We are taught to be careful but don't fully realize these things exist until it happens. It happens and we can't take it back. I never thought it would happen to me. I turn off the faucet of cold running water. I avoided my own reflection as I climbed back into bed. Tears distorted my vision. I felt *broken*. I had fallen apart. My chest hurt and it was hard to breathe. This was a level of selfishness I could never fully understand.

"I just wanna move on with my life, man!" He yelled at me as he grew tired of arguing.

How unfair of him to say when his actions would affect me for the rest of mine. One of my girl friends had lain beside me. The days pass. Her eyes dim with sorrow as she watched me become removed from reality. It must have been incredibly difficult for her to witness her friend so immensely distraught. I lose track of time and the mood swings, the mood swings make me want to scream.

In an ideal world, he would show true remorse for his actions without trying to justify them. In this world, that was more than he was willing to give. "What do you want from me?! You want me to caress you? Hold you? I'm not your fucking boyfriend!" He shouted over the phone.

"No, I don't want that!" I shouted back in disgust. It wasn't up for discussion whether or not he should be held accountable. I didn't know what to do. I thought back to our previous conversations. "I don't know what to say. I've had girls call me saying they're pregnant. Come to find out, there's more to it." I couldn't believe what I was hearing. He attempted to take the blame off of himself. I contemplated what I should do over the next few weeks. But my nightmare was far from over.

"You know this is wrong." My voice softened. The blame game. I wasn't entirely sure who was at fault. Myself or him. At first, I placed the blamed solely on my choice to have unprotected sex with a man who was not committed to me. If I hadn't slept with him, this wouldn't have happened. He convinced me I was the reason for his cruel entitlement. "You're trying to point fingers by not accepting responsibility for anything?! Like you're completely innocent," He said with sarcasm.

As if the conversation wasn't hard enough, he made it more difficult for the both of us. I could call him all the names in the book but I didn't. His defense hinted there could be more to *his* story. For days, I slept away the pain. I isolated myself completely. If I were around people, they would know something was different about me. That's what I thought at least. I imagined I had the H word stamped on my forehead.

The emotional toll was by far worse than actually living with the disease.

"It's just a virus. A skin condition," I told myself.

While this was true, it was to some degree inevitable; I didn't want to make it sound less than it was. I couldn't give it too much thought or power over me. If I don't think about it, it's not there.

*Denial.*

I messaged him frequently within the first month. It was no longer me he was talking to. My pain and suffering caused me to lash out towards him. A piece of me was gone and I wanted it back. My friend leaves me alone in her room to shower. I spent the entire time on her floor sobbing. The diagnosis left me in a confused daze. I sat for hours wishing I could erase every moment I had with him. Each time he touched me. From the first moment we met, to the last time we were intimate. I hate him. It wasn't his intention for things to spiral out of control.

At night, I was *rageful.* Tossing and turning in discomfort. I could feel a sharp sting like pins and needles poking at my skin. He failed to see that my experience differed from his. The transition is difficult for some. Like a newly awakened vampire eager to feed its thirst. I had a false sense of self. The part of me I thought was unbreakable; until I was bitten. My intent is not to be dramatic; rather to explain the transition people like me go through. I've been bitten. Although it's not fatal, I'm forever changed. The difference between him and I is risk. He believes with sex, comes risk. He says we should be adults about this. Take some time to calm down and speak to each other respectfully. We had several conversations within the next month. Most of them turned into a screaming match.

Afraid my friends and family would judge me or view me differently if they knew, I shut them out. I distanced myself from everyone. I ignored text messages and phone calls from those I loved most. I could feel myself losing grip of reality while I isolated for months.

*Anxiety.*

I sat on my bed staring at the label of my prescription. The walls of my room suddenly began closing in on me. I couldn't breathe. I screamed at the top of my lungs. I understood it was going to take time until I could find some light in the situation. His dishonesty threw me for a whirlwind of emotions. Who could I trust?

*Hopelessness.*

I saw no possibility of resuming back to a normal dating life. I had to remember who I was before my diagnosis.

My first day back to work was a blur. Walking into the building, I could hear my heart pounding. My palms were sweating. I wore a hat just low enough to cover my puffy eyes and dark circles from lack of sleep; anything to conceal my state of mind. I wasn't sure how to handle this. My college years were taking an unexpected turn.

I spent most of the day hiding out in nearby restrooms hoping no one would notice I was gone. I attempted to control my emotions but lost it each and every time. I sat against the toilet in a fetal position crying. The mood swings came in waves. I did look forward to my afternoon commute since it was the only time I wasn't expected to engage with anyone. My diagnosis hit hard due to lack of education surrounding the virus, my body's delayed responses and in the deceitful way it was acquired. In my mind, there was no distinction between the virus itself and betrayal. I couldn't separate the two.

It was explained to me about a year later that during this time, I had majorly disassociated and developed an adjustment disorder as well as anxiety. The body's natural trauma response is an attempt to remove oneself from a painful situation. How misplaced I felt. During lunch, I began researching the subject online. If this was going to be a part of me now, I might as well understand it. I couldn't stop thinking about what he had done to me.

Suddenly, the itch was back. And this time, it was accompanied by tiny red bumps. I was disgusted with myself and felt trapped in my own body. The tiny sores appeared minor in comparison to an average razor burn. But knowing exactly what this was somehow intensified it. My colleagues asked if I was ok when I returned. I felt obligated to say yes. So, I nodded and did just that. All while wondering how many of them were like me.

At first, it felt like the flu. I was fatigued and groggy. My immune system had been compromised as I finished an antibiotic treatment for bronchitis days before seeing him. My symptoms were ongoing, causing frequent outbreaks and infection until I developed antibodies. It was disheartening to learn there isn't an accessible cure. The sores would come and go throughout my lifetime, becoming less and less bothersome. I took a variety of supplements in order to avoid medication. He recommended dietary options in order to keep the virus under control. He must have been out of his mind to think I would consider taking advice from him. Each time the bumps reappeared, brought back the emotions. The agonizing pain lasted for days on end until my body was able to fight back.

*Regret.*

I wasn't entirely at fault. He should have said something. I trusted too easily and *that* was my mistake.

Throughout the first month, I walked the Brooklyn Bridge to my college campus after work. It was a form of release. I found peace in wandering from one borough to another. Tall buildings sprayed with the occasional graffiti tag surrounded the bridge. There was something alleviating about being so high off the ground. Far away from anyone who knew what had happened. I admired the East River through a large hole in the gate.

The sound of subway trains passing by was enough to drown out my screams at the top of the bridge. I inhale and exhale. I gazed at the waves as they splashed onto rocks by the highway. The hot sun beamed down on me, I knew I needed to end my despair. I wanted nothing more than to plummet to the bottom of the ocean. I didn't want to be alive. But I knew it wasn't the answer.

Suicidal thoughts were all I could think to alleviate my pain.

Would he understand the extent of my suffering if I take my own life?

Maybe then he wouldn't dare put someone through this again. "You're still the same person. This does not define you," my friend comforted me over the phone.

He spoke to me for hours every day until I was able to care for myself again.

"It could happen to anyone," his kind words struck a chord in my mind. I didn't think this was possible. I didn't think it would happen to *me*. "There's a lot of people that have it," my friend added.

*Acceptance.*
I was forced to learn how to love who I was all over again. After years of healing old wounds, I was left with another. "This doesn't change you. Don't let it get the best of you." I was reminded to continue on with life despite how hopeless I felt in the moment. The more I shared my secret with people close to me, the more I realized I wasn't alone.

It's common. Most of us don't talk about it. It's private. Some of us are afraid we'll be judged. Then there are others who fear rejection due to the stigma. The rest strongly believes in maintaining one's privacy. Each experience differs. Our stories are uniquely our own. Our "givers" vary from family members to someone we know and trusted. He is now considered mine. In some cases, it's impossible to learn who it came from. I had to forgive. Not considering the person who recklessly put me at risk for his own benefit, but myself for putting so much trust in him. It wasn't supposed to end this way.

"Just take the fucking pill! It's not the end of the world," he urged.

So, why did it feel like it was?

I refused to become dependent on antiviral medication for the rest of my life. I found eating specific foods triggered my outbreaks more than others. I was desperate to make them stop. I had trouble affording such a strict diet on my own. To ask the person responsible for help was degrading. My diet became restricted and natural supplements were expensive. Without antibodies, my body's natural defense against the virus was nonexistent. I felt I had no one else to turn to except him. He sent money electronically to help pay for my groceries. All I had to do was ask. He wasn't the ideal person to ask for help and I didn't want to speak to him. But wasn't sure who I could turn to. I called my mom who resides out of state more often than usual, praying her intuition would lead her to suspect something was wrong. I needed her. I wanted nothing more to do with him.

The blisters come in small clusters. And they aren't always painful. They resembled a paper cut or razor bumps. My fingers gently traced around them while I showered. I was careful not to touch them. I rinse the soap bubbles off of my skin. Flashbacks to when I asked him when was the last time he got tested for STDs.

"Six months ago," was his answer.

I assumed he tested negative since I wasn't given anything further. Tears fall together with droplets of water. I watch them disappear into the shower drain. I didn't choose for this to happen. Some of us gave consent prior to contracting the virus.

*Bitterness.*

From my fingers to my feet, nerve impulses became more frequent. I'm uncomfortable in my own skin. The blisters burst, leaving light stains on my underwear. I should've never allowed him to touch me. Regardless of our casual relationship, I am still a human being.

I step out of the shower wrapping my body in a bath towel. I think back to the time when I felt sexy in my bare skin. Not now. Not ever. I didn't think it would be possible to feel that way again. As I get dressed, I replay our conversations.

"You contacted me, you wanted it," He accused. His voice exuded guilt.

"You contacted me too!" I yelled back. "Yeah? Well not as often as you. I have the messages,' he said.

His apologies felt empty. Sorry wasn't enough. I remembered asking on more than one occasion if he wanted to stop seeing each other. Never did he say yes. He would apologize then make time to see me as soon as he could. Suddenly, I was the one who wanted this from the beginning.

## Chapter 2

# HIM

⌒

He was an attractive business man working as a director of marketing for two major clubs in Manhattan. Known for their strict door policy and elite clientele, they were often a topic of discussion for NYC's night goers. The popular clubs were considered two of New York City's hot spots. Almost everyone I knew partied at both venues. I was working as a hostess at a trendy restaurant in Midtown. It was a modern steakhouse with an upscale lounge and DJ booth. The ambience provided guests with a club-like atmosphere. An elegant fireplace stood out front behind tinted glass doors. He was a guest who came in on occasion for business. Marketing and management seemed to be his forte. Dressed in a suit, he was accompanied by beautiful women.

At the time, I had very little interest in boys my age. They were often immature, lost, and full of uncertainty. I preferred mature, mysterious men. I failed to realize maturity isn't measured by age but from mindset. Fifteen years my senior, I was just twenty-one when we met. With a youthful spirit and vibrant smile, his aura was warm and inviting. His skin, fairly smooth with very little facial hair. Dark, almond shaped eyes grew tired as they were slightly wrinkled at each corner. I found our age difference enticing. There was something about being in the presence of an older man.

Daddy issues.

The most heartbreaking experience a girl can have. It led to a distorted view on sex and relationships. I spent years trying to fill a void only a father's love could fulfill.

"Could you show these gentlemen to the table?" My coworker signaled over to their designated section.

I walked guests over to the dining area one by one. A couple sat in one of the booths with black leather seats surrounded by yellow and white lilacs. The restaurant's modern decor consisted of a soft yellow highlighted with black accents. The DJ could be heard playing a variety of hit music and top 40s. The restaurant itself was suitable for all ages. Employees were encouraged to keep the party going during busy hours. We'd dance in the center of the lounge with guests while music played. I glanced down at the time on the computer screen at the host stand. My feet swelled from standing in two inch heels all night. As the restaurant emptied, I noticed a man sitting alone by the bar engaged in conversation with the cocktail waitress.

His suit perfectly tailored. It accentuated his broad shoulders and tall physique. His short brown hair styled to compliment his relatively handsome facial features. He was sharp and dressed to impress. His charm welcomed conversation. With bright eyes and strong jawline, he exuded an overly confident demeanor. I had a weakness for tall business men in suits.

My attraction to him was almost instant. The way he composed himself was quite appealing. Our eyes locked from across the dining room. I craved being touched by the hands of a man. There was something about him that drew me to him. He possessed a strong, masculine sexual energy. A man of presence, I had to know who *he* was.

I could feel him watching as I made my way over to the cocktail waitress. A little, black dress tightly hugged my curves. I imagined his hand slowly sliding up the slit of my dress. It was said that men who worked nightlife had awful reputations. In the event you were lucky to find one that wasn't a playboy, it could possibly work in your favor. I asked the cocktail waitress about him from behind the bar. They seemed familiar with one another. She informed me he was a regular who worked closely with one of the managers.

I was intrigued as she didn't seem to know much else about him. As I headed downstairs to the coat room, I looked over at him and smiled. He followed a few steps behind as I pretended not to notice. I grabbed a yellow ticket from the coat check, carefully locking the door behind me. The stairs which led back to the main dining room were just past the restrooms. I hurried back to the host stand before management could take notice. On his way to the men's room, he stopped to gain my attention. This was the first time we spoke.

"I like your necklace," he complimented a silver rhinestone choker I was wearing.

"Why haven't I seen you before?" He asked for my name.

"I started working here a few months ago." I said.

He introduced himself by handing me a business card. His first and last name, along with contact information were displayed in small letters along with the company he worked for. He suggested I stop by one of the clubs sometime. At the time, I wasn't into the party scene.

"Are you even twenty-one?" He smirked.

My petite figure frequently made me mistaken for younger than my actual age. I assumed he was attempting to recruit me to work for him.

"I just turned twenty-one in August. Are you trying to take me out of this place?" I asked.

"I'm trying to take you for myself," he answered.

My mind filled with ideas as to how he would put his words into actions.

I hadn't been intimate with anyone in almost a year. The sexual tension heightened as his brown eyes fixated on me. He had a look of intensity like he wanted to devour every inch of my body. And I wanted him to. Due to his age, I wondered if he was secretly married or had any children. When he gave me his business card, I peeked at his ring finger. There were no indications of a wedding band.

Married men frequently came to the restaurant in search of eye candy or accompanied by their mistresses. Young women like myself were viewed as the target for emotionally unavailable men. We were considered naive. And although these men were never fully accessible to the women they so eagerly chased, it was almost always about control.

Back on the main dining floor, the manager awaited me with a smile. "So, what do you think of my boy?" He asked in curiosity. "He's cute," I said, trying not to blush. "Did you guys have a chance to talk?"

He stood beside me as we thanked each guest for coming as they exited. "He gave me his card."

Why?" I hesitated.

"He asked about you. He said you were beautiful and wanted to know who you were. I said you're one of the new hostesses and gave him your name," He explained.

"Whatever happens between you two, I want you to know that I only know him from here."

It seemed they knew each other from a business standpoint. "We've never hung out outside of work or anything like that," my manager warned.

A tall man with women wrapped around each of his arms approached the host stand.

"Text me," he winked on his way out. I watched the group exit the restaurant. He called for car service while the girls took pictures out front. His job required him to market some of NYC's major nightlife destinations. I was still healing the wounds of my last relationship. I wanted someone I could enjoy myself with for the time being. I sent him a text message shortly after his departure. He asked when I would be able to come to one of the clubs. I wasn't into his gesture and suggested he take me out on a date instead.

To which he replied, "When are you free?" This way, we could get to know each other more. He was a sweet talker, flirtatious by nature. I agreed to go out to dinner with him this upcoming Sunday.

His schedule was hectic. We hardly spoke the following week. He sent a chain message wishing me a Happy Cinco de Mayo. It was becoming clear he had no intention to get to know me.

"He's probably waiting until we see each other at dinner," I attempted to make sense of his distant behavior, overlooking what bothered me. I believed a man who truly wanted to get to know me would make an effort to keep conversation despite our plans. My replies shortened and his messages went unanswered. He quickly took notice.

"Hey! I'm having dinner at your job. I don't see you here," he messaged. He stopped by the job spontaneously. On each occasion, I was working part time at another restaurant. Except one.

The outside patio filled with guests and neon lights coming from the bar.

"Guess who just texted me?" My manager laughed.

I assumed it was *him*. He arrived with two blonde women and showed them to the main bar located inside the restaurant. Shortly after getting their drinks; he made his way over to the patio.

"Hey! Why haven't you texted me back?" He questioned immediately.

"I'm not really into texting, I prefer phone calls," I said. While this was technically true, I didn't want to say I was bothered by his inconsistent text messages. "Oh? I'll make sure to give you a call then. Are you looking forward to Sunday?" He smiled.

"Are you?" I diverted the question to avoid sounding overly excited. His impression of just wanting sex from me was a turn off.

"I'm looking forward to it." He nodded, paying close attention to the details of my outfit. "I like your boots." He never failed to comment on what I was wearing. He wasn't a man of details but he did have an eye for what looked appealing. He asked if I'd eaten before, insisting on ordering something from the menu. "I can't, I'm working." I said. "So?" He shrugged off my concern. His self-assurance was admirable. "Surprise me," I suggested he choose his favorite item. "How do you feel about dessert?"

A few minutes later, he brought over a to-go bag and left it for me at the host stand. Inside, was a freshly made cheesecake. I walked over to him gently placing my hand on the middle of his back. "That was sweet of you. Thank you." I smiled.

"It only gets better," he said.

He was charming. A smooth talker yet careful with his words.

"What about the girls you came with? Shouldn't you be getting back to them?" I teased him by referring to the women he left at the bar.

"I'm actually working right now...I don't want you to get jealous." He joked flirtatiously. I saw no reason to compete for someone's attention and felt the need to make that clear to him. Our eyes met when I responded back to his comment, "I don't get jealous. I just watch. I observe." The physical attraction between us was hard to ignore. It is from my understanding that lust can be just as blinding as love. I disregarded the nuances of his character. I wanted him to want me. Seduction at its finest.

When Sunday arrived, I thought he had forgotten about our date. I didn't hear from him until later that evening. My phone rang as I didn't have a signal and the call was sent to voicemail.

"Hey beautiful, just checking in to see if we're still on for dinner. If not, let me know so I can go ahead and arrange other plans. Give me a call back babe, bye." I returned his call then raced home to get dressed. He presented me with two restaurants to choose from. One with a gorgeous view, the other promoted plant based food choices. I previously mentioned my interests in health and wellness. It was nice to see he took it into consideration. I went with the one with the best view as it would be ideal for a date. Dinner required conversation and I was unsure how it would go.

He said he would call me a cab and when it arrived, I rushed out the door. A familiar face greeted me. "Are you Destiny?" The driver asked. The back seat could be seen through the mirror. I took a second look as he removed his hat. He drove from Manhattan to the far end of Brooklyn to surprise me and pick me up himself. "You're too cute!" I said moving to the passenger seat. We talked about our jobs, families, places we've lived and what led him to working nightlife. But there was one thing was weighing on my mind. "I have a question," I paused.

"Are you married? Any kids?" I looked at him eagerly awaiting his answer. "No," he said. "I've been fortunate enough not to have any kids. But I do have younger siblings. I guess you can say they're kind of like my kids."

On the way there, his father called in. They spoke briefly while he drove. I could tell he cared deeply for his family. I then learned he was just getting out of a five year relationship. "We live together," he mentioned. "Well, she lives with me but she's moving out soon," he explained further. "She's looking for a place."

I can empathize with the difficulty of a break up. I was glad he was honest with me about her. "Are you okay with each other dating? It must be awkward living together doing your own thing." I asked. "My ex and I have lived together and dated other people. I don't know what she's doing now but we don't need to talk about that," he said. He went on to say how much he respects her. His honesty only made him more attractive. I took his word for their relationship status and trusted he would tell me if there was anything else I should be aware of. The conversation flowed, he was very easygoing.

Our table was small and intimate, with a view of the East River. The city lights of Manhattan reflected off the dark water.

"The view is so beautiful!" I exclaimed. "So is mine," he said beaming from across the table through the candle light. As a dedicated business man, he traveled for work. After moving to New York City from the south a few years back, he became a nightlife guru. He made me laugh, and remained playful throughout the night. We skipped dessert and headed to an underground comedy club in Soho. "Oh my god it's cold," I shivered as the wind blew my hair. He took off his jacket and placed it over my shoulders as we walked to the car. A southern gentleman.

He held me by my waist on our way to the venue. I noticed the more drinks he had, the bolder he became. We were greeted by a security guard asking for an entree ID. The place was small and discreet. He ordered us drinks. I rested my leg on top of his as I watched the show. He ordered nachos and started to unwind. I declined alcoholic beverages choosing to stay sober for the night. The stand up comedians were engagingly hilarious. I felt his lips gently kiss my right shoulder. His hand carefully slid down my waist and into my skirt. He firmly squeezed the side of my naked thigh. I wanted to say something but I couldn't. The slightest touch aroused me. His face focused on the performance while his hand worked its way to my inner thigh. I excused myself to the restroom to stop him from going further. When I got back, he slipped his hand back into position and left it for the remainder of the show. The temptation was hard to ignore.

We walked to a shop across the street for a late night snack after the show. "I'm gonna need a kiss to seal the second date," he pulled me in aggressively. His body language signaling for a kiss. A gentle tap, I then pushed him away. "That's all you get for now," I said. It was only a kiss, but it felt rushed. "If she wasn't there I would've invited you back," he said referring to his ex-girlfriend. It was our first time out together. I wasn't looking to jump into bed so soon. "And what would we do if I went back with you?" I asked sarcastically. "What do you think?" He responded. "Who said I would go back with you anyway?" I asked in offense. "I can extend the invitation but you do not have to accept," he explained. Fair enough.

We talked for a bit waiting for a car to take me home. When it arrived, he opened the door for me to get in. "Have a goodnight babe. Get home safe," he said before kissing me on the lips. On the way home, I received a text message from him, "I had fun with you tonight. Can't wait until next time." It was then that I was certain he wasn't interested in anything more than a "good time." Not that I hadn't done it before, but part of me felt uncomfortable sleeping with someone I hardly knew. Another part of me wanted to.

A few days later, he wished me a good week as I didn't respond to his previous message. I decided to tell him what was on my mind. I felt he was being too forward. I wanted us to enjoy the moment and take things slow. "I respect you. I will be honest I'm getting out of a five year relationship looking to have fun right now. I don't want to give you the wrong idea," he said. "Most guys will tell you what you want to hear," he said. Like him, I wasn't looking for a relationship anytime soon. I did however, want to be careful with who I slept with in which I explained. "Let's enjoy getting to know each other for now," I continued. "Sounds good. We will when I get back," he replied with a kiss. "Have a safe flight," I said.

I didn't hear from him for months. At the time, I was unaware he was tying up loose ends with an ex girlfriend. It was clear we were on complete different pages when it came to sex.

As much as I wanted to sleep with him, I preferred us to wait. During an afternoon shift at the restaurant, my manager informed me he was back in town. "So is he going to fly you out one of these days?" He asked regarding future business trips. "I don't know. He hasn't contacted me," I shrugged. Another sign went overlooked. "Hope all is well," I reached out to him once. Then again three months later, for my 22nd birthday.

# Chapter 3

# THE GREEN DRESS

It would be one of the most important nights of my life. It would be one that would spark the beginning to an end. The beginning of a new chapter in my life and an end to the old me. Finding the perfect venue to celebrate my upcoming birthday was anything but easy. I was working two jobs in order to make ends meet. I overheard one of my coworkers discussing her drunken nights at the nightclubs he worked for. Although we hadn't spoken since our date, I decided to reach out via text message. Perhaps we could set something up for the occasion.

To my surprise, he responded promptly agreeing to help celebrate. He would take care of the table and venue asking for nothing in return. During the week, I gave him a call to make sure we were still on for the weekend. We proceeded to discuss further details.

I recall he did mistake the dates of the party. Resulting in our first disagreement. In the end, everything came together perfectly.

A small group of friends and I got ready for the night. I slipped into a beautiful, silk green dress. Its lightly colored fabric glimmered in the moonlight. Gently wrapping along the left side of my hip, exposing my upper thigh. It's plunged neckline exposes the sides of my breasts through its thin, silk detail. I wore metallic gold heels in addition to the appeal of the dress. I felt radiant. "What are you going to do if he invites you back to his place?" My girlfriends assumed he'd give it another try. "I don't think he's going to. He's working," I doubted. "If he does, I'll go. But only if he asks," I laughed. It was my birthday night. I should enjoy myself to the fullest, right?

Loud beats could be heard from outside the club. There was a line of men and women waiting to get in. Security heavily guarded the front entrance. "Destiny!" He shouted, waving at us to skip the line. "How many?" He asked. "Just three for now. The rest are on their way." I said. The security guard asked each of us for identification. He brought us inside where he suggested two areas for my table. One by the main entrance, the other in a VIP section next to the stage. He looked just as handsome as I remembered. The club was dark with very little lighting. A fluorescent sign with bright pink letters stood out against the wall.

Silver and black balloons awaited me at the table. He brought over tequila shots to get the party started. "Cheers to the birthday girl! Happy birthday!" Everyone shouted. Another round of shots followed. The club filled rapidly with crowds of people on the dance floor. "Make sure she doesn't go anywhere," he whispered to one of my guy friends. Sparklers and a birthday cake were sent over to surprise me while I was in the restroom. Bottle girls danced around the table holding the cake in the air. When I got back, I caught the tail end of it. "Thank you," I kissed him on the cheek. Two bottles of champagne and vodka sat in the center. Orange and cranberry juice were presented as mixtures. Everyone was completely drunk by the end of the night.

"Dance with me!" I shouted at the busser. "I can't Miss, I am working!" he laughed. I stumbled over to the couch to pour myself another drink. I accidentally knocked over champagne glasses as I sat down. My friends and I laughed it off, dancing the night away. The smell of cigar smoke oozed out from behind a red curtain in the back room. Two mainstream artists performed as the crowd gathered around the DJ booth. I climbed on top of a nearby couch to gain a better view. "Do you want champagne?!" A young woman handed me another glass before I could say yes. During the performance, I looked for him in the crowd. I saw him pacing back and forth through the club managing the floor as he spoke into his headset.

I moved my hips to the beat of the music. My dress swayed with every movement. He snuck up behind me. "You look sexy in that dress. That side boob has my attention," he whispered into my ear.

"Oh, you've been looking?" I giggled. "Of course I have!" He admitted without hesitation. "You look handsome yourself," I complimented. He must've picked up on the sexual tension as he wasted no time getting straight to the point. "Do you want some birthday sex?" He leaned in closer. The amount of alcohol I consumed had no effect on my decision. I had assessed the outcome of leaving with him before I arrived. I nodded "Yes." And gave my consent. He asked that I wait for him while he immediately began closing down for the night.

"I never leave this early," he said, taking my hand as we headed towards the exit. Waiting out front, my friends asked for his business card in case of emergency. I stumbled beside him waiting for a cab. He buckled his motorcycle helmet. "Why can't I get on?"

I asked drunkenly.

"I only have one helmet," he said.

"I'm sending you in a car behind me."

A black Honda parked next to the street curb. "Get in. I'll meet you there," he said, helping me shove balloons into the backseat. He shut the door and got on his motorcycle. Blurred red and yellow street lights passed as I placed my head against the window. He called to direct the cab driver to drop me off at the back entrance of his house. It was a private community with a gateway entry.

He assisted with keeping my balance as we walked upstairs. The apartment was a spacious three bedroom. Warm neutral colors blended into the dark wooden furniture. I followed him down a small hallway leading to the master bedroom. "Aren't you going to give me a tour?" I asked peeking into the rooms. I pushed the door open and was able to see inside the first. There was no furniture, no artwork, it was empty. "I'm renting it out. Someone should be moving in soon," he said. I dropped my balloons to the floor, held together by a paper weight. Behind the next door was a king sized bed covered in dark sheets. The lighting was dim and sensual. I took off my heels and laid down spreading my arms across the bed. The ceiling began to spin. I could hear music by my favorite artist playing in the background.

He stood over me at the edge of the bed tugging at the green dress.

"Now let's get this off you," he said, helping me to undress. "No panties," he smirked, revealing I was naked underneath. His lips caressed mine. He kneeled down, opening up my legs in front of his face. There was nothing I enjoyed more than a man who wasn't afraid to please a woman in ways he would want for himself. I moaned tightly gripping onto the sheets, my back arching upward. Licking me until I was ready for him to intrude. He used his fingers first, leading up to penetration. I stopped him. "Do you have a condom?" I sat up breathing heavily. Despite my drunkenness, I somehow remembered the saying, "safety first."

He opened a drawer by the night stand anxiously unwrapping a latex condom. I pulled him in closer, kissing his neck as he struggled to put it on. My nails dug into his shoulders as I held onto his arms. He squeezed my breasts before placing them in his mouth. I could feel him moving deeper and deeper. He let out a soft groan before turning me over. My long, dark hair wrapped around his fist while he entered me from behind. My muscles weakened as he penetrated me. Now face to face, he instructed me to say, "thank you," for taking care of me on my birthday night. I loved the way he felt.

His large body laid back as I straddled him. "Yes Destiny!" He shouted my name in excitement, holding me by my hips. As I took control, I looked down to find the condom was gone. We engaged in rough, passionate sex until sunrise. I was caught in the moment. And at that moment, there were no repercussions. The sun peeked through the windows of his bedroom, our bodies pressed together drenched in sweat. Each time he finished, it was from behind. He couldn't seem to have it any other way. I glanced up at the clock, his arm wrapped around me as we laid naked.

"Goodnight," I said softly stroking the hairs on his arm. "Goodnight babe," he held me tightly as eyes began to shut.

*Detachment.*

Something we had in common. I woke up to find him still asleep beside me. The green dress and heels were scattered over the bedroom floor. I searched for my phone to message my friends and let them know I was safe. My head was pounding from the hangover. They were happy to hear about our rendezvous. He awoke to the sound of my voice discussing the rest of my plans over the phone.

"Good morning," I smiled.

"Good morning babe," he managed to open his eyes for a split second.

"I think I'm ready to go," I said, hanging up the phone.

"Okay. I will call you a cab. But first…one more time before you go birthday girl." He pulled me in for another round. Morning sex.

"Did you have fun?" I searched the room for my bra. "I did. You have a filthy mouth! I thought you were innocent," he said laying in bed. I couldn't remember much of what was said the night before.

"Well, you're not going to know everything about me after one date," I responded swiftly to his assumption. "I see," he said, scrolling through his phone checking for emails. He climbed out of bed to walk me downstairs. "Ah, the walk of shame," he joked. I never felt it was a wrong for a woman to have casual sex if that's what she chooses. Nevertheless, this was a strange concept to some. "I'm not ashamed. I don't regret anything," I said. It was a birthday well spent.

"Take care babe. Enjoy the rest of your day," he held the cab door open and kissed me goodbye.

Later that day, I shared some of the erotic details with my girlfriends at brunch. His scent lingered on my skin. I considered keeping him around for sex. After all, I did enjoy it. If I wanted to keep this going, I would have to be upfront with him.

"Thank you for everything. I had a great time. I wouldn't mind doing it again," I said over the phone. He laughed and we agreed to keep in touch. That weekend, I contacted him after gaining some liquid courage. When I wanted something, I was determined to get it.

"Heyyyyy!" He replied to my text message.

"I'm drunk," I laughed. "Already? It's too early!" He replied. "What time do you get off work?" I asked.

"Not until late. Text you when I'm on my way home," he said. I received a message from him around 5:00 am. "Send address so we can play," it said. From Brooklyn to Manhattan, he sent cabs in the middle of the night that brought me to his place. I watched the sunrise over behind tall buildings along the highway. We lived about 40 minutes from each other.

"How far are you?" He messaged again. "About 20 minutes due to traffic," I replied.

He responded impatiently, "I'm falling asleep."

It had only been a few days since we last saw each other. "You're in big trouble for making me wait," He said. I suggested he punish me as I waited for traffic to subside. Walking up the pathway to his building, I saw him standing outside in a hoodie and sweatpants smoking a cigarette. He greeted me with a kiss. "How was work?" I asked.

"It was hectic tonight." He grabbed me by my back end and smacked it. When we got upstairs, I was alarmed when I discovered my time of the month came early. I explained it was unexpected but he didn't believe me.

"Look. I've been around the block. You don't have to lie to me. Women are the horniest on their periods." I was taken aback by his shameless remarks. "Do you even have a tampon with you?

I guess you're going to have to give a lot of head." He laid back waiting for me to get to it.

If this was part of my punishment for making him wait, he was being an asshole about it.

"Should I leave?" I asked irritably.

"You're already here babe," he said, adjusting himself. I proceeded to do as I was told. How heavy is your period?" He asked me to show him. Despite only being intimate for the second time, he seemed oddly comfortable despite the circumstances. "Oh, that's nothing," He said opening my legs. I could feel his erection against me.

"Ouch! It hurts!" I yelled as he intruded without a condom.

"It hurts?" He asked, positioning me. "Yeah," I moaned. "Shut up," he commanded in an aggressive tone. He continued punishing me, forcing me into a half split. Later, I felt him speed up and suddenly pull out.

He grabbed a towel to wipe us off. Soothing nature sounds filled the room with tranquility. These were the sounds we would fall asleep to each night we spent together. "I can't feel my legs," I told him. "Let's get to bed. I feel bad now that I hurt you," he laid down beside me. "It's okay. I liked it," I rolled over and fell asleep with his arm around me. A couple hours later, I awoke to him touching me inappropriately. But I didn't want him to stop. "I thought we were going to sleep," I said. "We are." He spanked me again while pressing me down against the bed. I lay on my stomach watching our shadows move along the bedroom walls.

The next morning, I left uncertain if it would be the last time we saw each other. It wasn't. For the next seven months, we met on and off when he was in town. I worked during the day, he worked nights. Our work schedules were completely opposite. We did what we could to make it work. "Where are you?" He asked.

"Do you want to come over?" He offered to call me a cab. Still half asleep, I quickly got out of bed to fix my hair and apply light makeup. Our hookup times were usually spontaneous and unexpected. It was exciting sneaking off into late hours of the night. The city that never sleeps. When I got there, he sat me on top of him as he began fondling me.

# Chapter 4

# PAIN AND PLEASURE

⟶

My face muffled into a pillow case. The bed frame pounded against the wall matching the rhythm of his thrusts.

"We probably woke up my neighbors," he said trying to catch his breath.

"At least they know your name now," I joked.

"Agua?" He handed me a jar of water he kept by the nightstand. I laid beside him, my leg gently resting on top of his.

"Move over," he told me as he carefully inspected the bedsheets.

"Well that's a first," he sighed. My nails must've accidentally torn through the fabric.

"Between sex and the cat these sheets aren't going to last," he said before lying down. His cat jumped into bed purring as it crept onto my lap. Its green eyes pierced mine before running off again in search of food. I pulled the covers up to my bare chest with my lower back slightly pressed against him. "No mas," he said as he began piling blankets and pillows to build a small barrier.

"Did you really just build a wall between us?" I laughed peeking over its thin layers. "Yes. I need to get some rest, babe," he closed his eyes. I looked over at the closet door. I wasn't satisfied just yet.

A collection of silk ties, collared shirts, and belt buckles could be seen dangling from inside. Baseball caps hung over the wooden door frame and a small workout trampoline sat by the wall. "You should tie me up with one of your belts," I suggested. His eyes opened.

"I can wake up for that," he said, making his way over to the closet. I watched him. He selected a fabric belt for us to use.

"Lie down." He commanded. My arms and legs were then tied in a knot.

"Not too tight," I uttered.

"You're such a naughty girl," he said hovering over me. It was aggressive and rough. It was a pleasurable kind of pain. I was tossed around like a rag doll, submissive to his liking. Eventually, my ankles were untied as I performed without the use of my hands. He then untied my wrists. In due time, I developed a sense of trust in him. He made me feel safe; chest to chest, my legs wrapped around his waist. I pulled him in closer with each climax. By the end, we were covered in sweat. "Okay, that's enough for tonight," he grabbed a towel from the back of his desk chair. Our poor use of protection caused me to question his actions outside of our friends with benefits relationship.

"We need to get better at using condoms," I mentioned. "Are you going unprotected with other people?" I became suspicious of him as it pertained to my health. I felt it was more than appropriate to discuss whether or not he was having unprotected sex with other women. Lack of protection meant I was susceptible to countless diseases he could possibly transmit.

"That's none of your business missy." He answered rudely.

"You don't see me asking questions." His dismissive response did not sit well with me.

By morning, I'd forgotten about our conversation regarding safer sex. "Baby, is it okay if I don't walk you down this time? I'm fucking exhausted," he asked laying under the covers. "I wonder why," I teased. "Well, *someone* kept me up all night," he said. While I understood he was running on very little sleep, I still cherished gentlemanly acts. "Here I go, walking myself to the door..." I looked back at him to show I wasn't okay walking myself out. "The things I do for you," he groaned as he got out of bed and walked me downstairs. "Get home safe," he opened the car door and leaned in for a quick kiss.

Two weeks passed. In the middle of the night, I received a text message. "Destiny come over," he wrote. I planned to see him at one of the clubs he worked for later that week for a girls' night out. "I'll see you Friday," I replied back. "What if I want to see you now?" He urged. I chose not to respond to his message before falling back asleep. There were times I wasn't up for it. We spoke again Friday night. My friends and I were just around the corner from the venue when I messaged him. I wore a see-through bronze cover up in the form of a dress along with a bodysuit. My outfit stood out from the rest.

I introduced him to my girlfriends before he walked us over to take shots by the bar. "Cheers!" We were given shot glasses and drink tickets. Following behind him, we were escorted to a table by the entrance used to promote the club. I unapologetically danced on the couch, colorful lights flickered over the checkered dance floor. I felt a hand firmly grip my backend. I turned around to find him walking passed me, pushing through the crowd as he talked into his headset. He flirted with discretion despite being on the job. It was an unspoken rule that whenever I came to the Manhattan night club, I would go home with him.

From a distance, I saw a young woman who worked as a bottle girl speaking closely with him, leaning into his ear. It would be of no surprise if she had slept with him too. The desire for a temporary distraction can be so strong we don't realize it. During the last hour, the dance floor began to empty. I sent him a message before leaving with my girlfriend. The club lights came on, signaling it was time to head home. "He didn't answer," I said to one of my friends as we waited for a cab.

"Do you think he's going home tonight with another girl?" I questioned, thinking of the young woman talking to him and her body language. "He's probably going to text you when he's done working. Don't worry about it. Our cab is here," said my friend, as we got into the car. The drinks were catching up to me. I respected his decision to do as he pleased but hoped for communication at the very least.

Back in Brooklyn, my friend and I got ready for bed. I thought my plans with him had fallen through. I began getting ready for bed. My phone rings.

"Hey! Where are you?" He asked. "I'm in Brooklyn spending the night at my friend's house," I glanced at the time to find it was almost 6:00 am.

"I thought we had an agreement babe," he said.

"I asked if you still wanted me to go back with you but you didn't answer," I explained.

We were now about an hour away from each other.

"You do realize I'm closing down the club tonight right? Are you still wearing that dress? You looked like a Vegas showgirl," he exclaimed.

"Is that a good thing?" I asked unsure of his comment never having been to Las Vegas.

"Of course it is! Send your address." A black car will be parked across the street from the house within minutes.

"I'm glad you liked it," I said, draping the dress over my knee. "Yes I do. It's sexy. Can't wait to get it off you," he admitted. I was equally anxious to get to his apartment. On the highway, I looked out the car window as tall buildings and bridges passed by. The city is wonderfully luminous at night.

He laid on his back.

"Sit on my face," he instructed me.

"I haven't showered. We're coming from the club. Are you sure?" I hesitated before straddling him.

"Well now you have me thinking," He said in frustration. I proceeded to position myself onto his face. I could feel his tongue and the facial hair he'd recently grown out brush up against me. I held onto the bed frame while he devoured me. I looked down at him. He hummed softly into me. The vibrating sensation of his lips felt amazing. Sex with him put me at ease. There were severe personal struggles I was harboring inside. I never said a word to him about any of it. We didn't share our private lives with one another. Our relationship was based on one thing and one thing only.

He traveled more often than I preferred. Usually, he was out of town on business.

"When are you coming back to New York?" I asked.

"In about 3 months," he replied.

This was the longest trip he'd taken since we started seeing each other. He flew back to his hometown to visit family for a couple of days before taking care of business.

"You have my number if you want to see me when you get back. Safe Travels." I sent along a kiss.

"I will most definitely. Thanks babe," he messaged back. I sent a couple flirty text messages while he was away. To my surprise, he kept his word and contacted me towards the end of his trip.

"I will be back Monday," he implied he wanted to hook up. In the few months he was gone, I stopped working my summer job as a hostess and found myself in need of another part time job. Although I could obtain one on my own, he worked closely with several owners of local restaurants. Some of which were his friends. I figured I'd ask if he could recommend me.

"What position are you looking for?" I sat down on top of him, placing his hands under my sweatshirt. He held onto my hips. I was much smaller than him in size.

"Where do you want to start? A lot of places want a couple years of experience. It's pretty competitive in Manhattan," he said.

"I'll start at the bottom I guess," I said poking fun at myself. "You're cute," he said looking at me.

"I don't know. Maybe I could try cocktail waitressing or bottle service," I twirled a thin chain he wore around my fingers. He told me about a friend of his who owned a nightclub and recently opened a new restaurant and lounge in the Lower East side.

Later that week, he introduced me to the owner via group message. They were best friends, more like brothers. I was scheduled to come in for an interview. I immediately got a job at the restaurant working nights as a cocktail waitress. It was a great opportunity for me to gain experience, network and make some extra money. I truly appreciated his help getting me the job. I was naive to think his help wouldn't come at a price. My new boss was a handsome older man. His recent engagement didn't stop him from flirting with lady staff members on numerous occasions.

"He's probably going to hit on you," he cautioned me about his overly personable friend. If my pay wasn't being affected, I wasn't concerned with his flirtatious ways.

Sometime around 2:00 am.

"You're being sensitive. I am sorry if I made you think I ignored your feelings. I am fun-loving. I like to joke around and be playful. Try not to take everything so seriously," he wrote. Our bickering was becoming more and more frequent. Selfish and entitled, his true character began to unravel. I'm sure you are questioning as to why I continued seeing him when all of the signs were there. My answer is simple. I'm flawed. I make mistakes. Majority of us have been guilty of ignoring the early signs of toxicity at one point or another. On numerous occasions, he was given the opportunity to change the course of things and chose not to.

"You're a brat. It's like everything has to be your way," I snapped at him. "Oh stop it," He said, shutting the door behind us. Nevertheless, we were able to put our differences aside. For the sake of sex, of course. Each argument ended in spine-chilling orgasms. I didn't refrain from using the occasional word "dickhead" to describe him when telling him off. "Your cab will be here in five minutes Princess," he mocked. I found his arrogance incredibly irritating. He continued scrolling through his phone.

That winter, a snow storm hit the city forcing schools and public transportation services to shut down for the day. Blizzard covered streets covered by piles of frozen snow on the hood of parked cars. What a better way to spend the snow day than in bed? I grabbed my phone from the dresser to message him. There was no point in beating around the bush. I asked if I could come over before shoving a pair of black fishnet stockings into my purse. It was time to spice things up a bit. As I waited by my front door, I felt a vibration in my back pocket.

"Cab cancelled. Let's save it for another time," his text message read. Already dressed and ready to go, I asked that he send another. The snow was making it difficult for cars to get out on the road. I called twice until I received a response. Was I only wanted at his convenience? It was supposed to be convenient for me as well. Seriously? You're mad because you got out of bed? I will send a cab to get you tomorrow.

He thought it was unnecessary for me to be upset with him.

Snowed in the following day, hours passed well into the evening. I messaged him angrily. It was frustrating dealing with his inconsistency.

"Never mind," I said in regards to our plans. He replied simply without question as to what angered me; which only upset me further. Our dynamic felt controlling. I shook my head and tossed my phone onto the bed. The next day, I received another text message.

"Let's try this again," He proposed. I set aside my agitation from the previous day and carried on with my sexual distraction. The sun was beginning to rise, light seeped through the curtains of my bedroom.

"Hey! The cab is on its way," He sounded quite lively over the phone considering what time it was.

"I'm still getting dressed. Give me a few more minutes," I said finishing up.

"You don't need makeup babe, you have natural beauty," he tried sweet-talking me. '

"Are you going to come here with a smile on your face? You've been giving me a lot of attitude lately," he said.

I waited to speak with him in person to discuss what was bothering me. A cab parked in front of my place moments later. When I got to his apartment, he addressed the issue before I could.

"You need to communicate more instead of saying never mind with that little attitude of yours," he suggested as it would help to diffuse future arguments. Talking to him came easy. We seemed to resolve conflict and our arguments never escalated. A mutual sense of comfortability developed between us as the months went by. Not once did he allow me to remain upset with him. His head locked into my neck as he moved deeper inside me. This was the closest his body had been to mine. My lips caressed his right ear. Face to face, my nails dug into his back. Mid way, I found myself wondering where this was headed. It wasn't a relationship nor did I want it to be. There was a certain thrill that came without knowing the exact destination. I did however, consider him a friend. My friend with benefits.

Ignorance was bliss. I assumed he'd take proper safety precautions when sleeping with other women to ensure his safety. He took exceptional care of himself. From his hygiene to his food consumption. Health and fitness were of major interests. The following week, I awoke to a phone call. Still half asleep, I sent the unknown number to voicemail. It rang again and again until I answered.

"Destiny where are you?" He asked.

"Hey, I'm sleeping," I mumbled.

"Come over," he demanded.

"I can't. I have to go to work soon. I'll see you another day." I tried reasoning with him.

"What do you need? A doctor's note? I can get you one if that's what you want," he insisted.

"Are you okay?" I asked.

"Yeah. Just come over," he persisted.

"I can't. I have bills to pay," I said.

"How much are your bills? I'll pay one," he said.

"No thank you. You're crazy! I'll see you another day," I declined.

"I got you a job missy. You owe me a proper thank you," he refused to take no for an answer.

"Okay. I said thank you. I have to go to work. I'll see you sometime this week," I declined his offer once again.

"I don't see what the issue is. I said I'll get you a doctor's note. What is so difficult about that? Maybe you don't have a job then," he threatened my opportunity at the restaurant before abruptly hanging up the phone.

I waited for a Brooklyn bound Q train on the outside platform. Nearly an hour later, I received another text message.

"I am waiting. I will make my offer one last time," he wrote. I boarded the train and sat by the window. The next time I saw him, he was acting strange.

"Open the door. I'm tired," I answered outside his front door completely unamused. His erratic behavior was of great concern to me. He opened the door just enough for me to see the side of his face.

"What's the password?" He joked again. When the door finally opened, I placed my phone down on the table to take off my shoes. He took it and ran off placing it in the middle of the hallway leading to his bedroom.

"You're gonna have to come get it," he taunted. There were many different versions of him. This one in particular, reminded me of a small child.

"What did you take?" I awaited his answer as it was becoming increasingly more obvious he wasn't sober. "I had a few drinks," he admitted. Moments later none of that mattered as my head rested on his bare chest. I could hear his heart beating faster than usual.

"I feel like you're holding back," I expressed to him.

"You think I'm holding back?" He reiterated.

"Yes. It's like you don't allow yourself to let loose completely with me," I elaborated.

"I know you have a wild side. There's a lot more to you than you show." He tightly gripped my upper thigh. I noticed he was struggling to fall asleep. Delicately placing my fingers on the sides of his forehead, I massaged him.

"Focus on the now and try to relax," I began moving my fingers in circular motion.

"That's very nice of you," he said, closing his eyes. A woman's intuition is never wrong. I stared at him curiously. I wondered what secrets he was hiding. Or who he was hiding from.

Dark shadows on the walls outlined our naked bodies. He was exceptional at everything he did. "Thanks for the instructions," he said. I knew just what I liked and what I wanted. He jokingly referred to me as "sex machine." A term he used to describe me on more than occasion. Unlike our previous encounters, he was unable to finish. As I adjusted my clothes and fixed my hair in front of the mirror, he slowly came up from behind and wrapped his arms around me.

"I'm getting turned on watching you get dressed," his brown eyes glistened while he looked at me through the mirror. We made our way over to the bed. He bent me over and pulled down my jeans continuously filling my body with ecstasy. And when it was over, I didn't want it to be. He made me feel wanted. Unfortunately as time went on, so did our disagreements. Although I usually spent the night at his place and left whenever I pleased.

"Your cab is downstairs," he said. His face glued into his phone responding to his unanswered emails and text messages. I thought if we could put our differences aside, I would be able to hold onto my distraction for just a while longer.

## Chapter 5

# THE GIFT THAT KEEPS ON GIVING

"How's it going at the restaurant?" He poured a glass of wine. "It's going," I said searching the room for my bra.

"You two look like you would be friends." Has he tried flirting with you?" Ironically, there had been one occasion his friend flirted with me inappropriately.

"He told me to take my clothes off while I changed into a cocktail dress," I recalled.

"What did he say? Hey baby take those clothes off?" He mimicked his friend's heavy accent before laughing it off. It was a strangely accurate impression.

"So did you?" He held a glass of Pinot Grigio for us to share. "Yeah I did!" I rolled my eyes in sarcasm.

"No! What kind of girl do you think I am?!" I asked.

"Hey, I don't mind sharing," he shrugged his shoulders. "What's mine is his. He's like a brother to me." We walked over to the kitchen and stood by the front door. "I wouldn't sleep with a friend of yours. That's not me. I like tall guys anyway," I said in reference to his height of 6 '2. "Sorry for him!" he smiled. "Save it for daddy."

A week later, the job he'd gotten me at the restaurant ended abruptly. After several failed discussions with management regarding lack of pay, it was time to part ways. I sent a brief text message thanking him for the opportunity. I never meant to leave on bad terms. Later that night, I came down with a fever accompanied by night chills. My body ached as I sweat through most of my clothes. I fixed myself a cup of tea. Herbal remedies always seemed to do the trick.

I grew extremely tired and decided to get some rest. By morning, I awoke to an itch in an uncomfortable location. When I scratched, I noticed a tiny bump on the right side of my labia. I took a look as it appeared harmless. Slightly raised above the skin. It resembled an ingrown hair, only smaller. No sign of infection other than slight stinging from scratching. Eventually, the pain worsened. I must have irritated it.

The lesion brushed up against my underwear as I walked. I limped over to the bathroom to urinate. It burned! I attempted to wipe clean, gently patting the area dry. Usually, a hair follicle can be seen at the center of an ingrown hair. I took a closer look. Mine did not. Razor burn perhaps? Water splashed onto the open lesion as I showered. I struggled to rinse the area without touching it. If I stood still long enough, the pain would temporarily subside.

What was once considered an everyday task gave me incredible difficulty. I squatted over the toilet seat to avoid stinging when using the restroom; bringing my chest entirely up to my knees. It was the only position I could sit comfortably in. The next day, I took an express train to the nearest urgent care where a medical professional would examine me.

"It's most likely viral," the doctor said, studying what seemed to be the beginning stages of a rash developing across my chest. "Let's examine you further so I can see this bump you are telling me about."

I changed into my hospital gown and undressed from the waist down. Taking a deep breath, I laid back nervously, my legs tightly clenched together.

"Okay, try to relax," she instructed.

"Have you ever had a herpes outbreak?" She took out a pair of latex gloves.

"What? No!" I exclaimed. I was horrified as to why she would ask such a question.

"It looks to me like ingrown hair. It's probably infected. Don't keep picking at it. Try not to wear tight clothing. You can self treat it at home by soaking in epsom salt or we can prescribe a cream for you to use. The cream will work much faster." She assured me healing would take place within a few days.

"If it doesn't, give us a call," she instructed the nurse to prepare my paperwork for discharge.

"Any questions?" I left her office relieved. My bump was nothing more than an ingrown hair. I had worked myself up over something so minuscule. I followed her instructions as soon as I got home. After all, doctors know best.

I remained in pain for the next couple of days. Something wasn't right. I decided to visit another urgent care to gain a second opinion.

"Have a seat, the doctor will be right with you," The nurse gently closed the door. I looked around the doctor's office. Pastel paintings of outdoor landscapes hung on the walls. I read instructional posters on how to wash your hands-correctly. I never did enjoy going to the doctor.

"Can you tell me a little more about the symptoms you're having?" She sat on her stool. Where do I start? "I'm going to take a culture by swabbing the lesion. It's going to sting a bit but try to bear with me."

Before I could respond, I felt a sharp sensation similar to pouring hydrogen peroxide over a fresh wound. I clenched my jaw. Placing one hand over my mouth, the other tightly gripped the edge of the exam table.

"We're going to send this over to the lab for testing. But by looking at it, I'm pretty sure it's herpes," she concluded. My stomach dropped. Did she say *Herpes*?! My heart sank into my chest. I could visibly see her mouth moving yet couldn't hear a sound. I struggled to refocus. I thought I was going to pass out.

"You should know that this is extremely common," The sound of her voice began to fade. I heard just enough to catch the tail end of her sentences.

"We can provide you with more information once your test results come back," she said.

"Do you have any questions, Destiny?" I sat up in disbelief.

"You can tell just by looking at it? Are you sure? Another doctor told me it was ingrown hair."

My instinct was to reject the harsh reality of what she was trying to tell me. I was in denial.

"I can't say for sure right now until your bloodwork comes back, but I've seen it enough times to know what it looks like. And your symptoms are..." She carried on.

Her voice turned mute. I hadn't slept with anyone who has herpes. I've never seen bumps on any of them. None of them showed symptoms. Then again, I never knew much about it other than what was available on the internet.

"We will give you a call when the lab has been completed. Do you have any more questions for me?" I shook my head no. This wasn't possible. I remained hopeful she made a mistake and my test would come back negative. I was reluctant to believe her because I've always gotten tested after unprotected sex. Probably more often than I should. I make sure to ask my partners if they've been tested as well. This can't be right. And yet she sounded so sure. I called a friend as soon as I left the facility and shared what the doctor had told me. He too remained hopeful my lab results would say otherwise. As I lay in bed that night, I couldn't stop thinking about what the second doctor had said. I researched online for more information and discovered the misconceived horrors of what I would endure for the rest of my life.

The images online appeared much differently from my lesion. Distorted photos of male and female genitalia were almost unrecognizable. It was as if someone hand picked the most dramatically revolting images they could find to represent herpes. My body looked completely normal other than one insignificant bump which healed within days just as the doctor said it would. My thoughts scattered.

Who gave this to me? Was it him? Or a previous partner? Awaiting the lab results was the longest nine days of my life. Some of the symptoms in women include: fever, flu-like symptoms, pain in legs, headache, fatigue, itching, tingling, and malaise. Men often show no symptoms. I slowly began coming to terms with the possibility of being herpes positive. I learned sores aren't always present and they may or may not reappear after the first outbreak. As the days went by, I discovered shocking statistics stating 90 percent of the general population carry a strand of herpes. Many of which are asymptomatic. Cold sores are the most prevalent. I was curious as to how many of us don't know we're carrying the same virus that causes genital sores.

I received a phone call at work from an unknown number. When answered, a doctor confirmed my test results were in. I was asked to stop by the clinic to pick them up. I assumed the worst as I hadn't been asked to come in before. I couldn't wait any longer so I rushed over to the nearest urgent care on my lunch break. My hands and legs were shaking. When I got there, I sat in the waiting room nervously. My name was called to step into the doctor's office shortly after. There was a TV on low volume and a chair for me to sit in. I heard light footsteps down the hall. Then a knock at the door.

"Come in," I permitted.

With a clipboard in hand, the doctor greeted me. I was introduced to the nurse who was assisting him.

"How are you feeling today?" He asked. I'd spent the last week and a half trying not to feel sorry for myself while learning more about a condition I could possibly have.

"Not very good," I answered. I wanted to be anywhere but there.

"So did they tell you?" The doctor took a seat.

"No," I hesitated.

"It came back positive." His facial expression matched the previous doctor who examined me and the nurse. The Herpes Simplex Virus (hsv) is a viral infection spread through skin contact. While there are several viruses pertaining to the Herpes Zoster, such as chicken pox and shingles, there are two strains responsible for sores located around the mouth and genitals. BOTH are transmittable in either region. The first strain, Oral herpes (hsv1), better known as cold sores, are blisters located at the mouth. Hsv1 may be contracted genitally through oral sex. I repeat, cold sores can be transmitted genitally. This is known as ghsv1.

Despite what you may have heard, contraction of either strain may occur with or without a visible sore. Oral infections or cold sores, most often occur in childhood. Genital herpes (hsv2) is the second strain. Sores develop in the genital region. They are the same in different locations. However, it is less likely for hsv2 to spread to the mouth. During an outbreak, the probability of transmission heightens greatly. Without an outbreak, our bodies periodically undergo a process called viral shedding. This occurs when the host cell of the infection reproduces and replicates. Eventually, it leaves the cell and we begin to "shed the virus."

Detecting herpes can be tough. Although I was screened for STDs, I had never been tested for herpes. Typically, these tests screen for diseases such as Chlamydia, Trichomoniasis, Gonorrhea, amongst a few others. Hsv, hpv, and hiv are not included in routine testing. There was no way I could have possibly known I was being exposed. The best way to detect exposure is by requesting a blood test. While this can be expensive for some, it provides the most efficiency. It was extremely disheartening to learn this information.

And now I'm sharing it with all of you. To help others become sexually empowered by gaining knowledge and better understanding STDs. None of us are immune to them. Unless you are experiencing the physical symptoms of an outbreak or showing visible sores as I did, you will most likely not be tested for herpes. I still strongly encourage everyone to practice safe sex and continue getting tested as it is crucial to know your status. If anyone would like more information regarding screenings, please do not hesitate to speak with your doctor or health care provider.

"Since this is your first outbreak, we are prescribing medication in case you have ongoing symptoms. Take them orally as needed," the doctor instructed.

"Have you started taking any of the medications from your previous visit?" Tears began to form as the nurse handed me a tissue.

"It's okay if you need to take a moment," he empathized.

"I can't." I anxiously smiled wiping away my tears. "I'm on my lunch break. I have to go back to work soon," The nurse handed me the entire box of tissue.

"So there's no cure for this, right?" I thought back to the numerous articles I had forced myself to read about hsv.

"As of right now, there is no cure but we can help minimize your outbreaks. They won't be nearly as painful or frequent as time goes on," he informed.

"And there's no way to know who gave this to me?" I crumbled up what was left of a tissue into the palm of my hand.

"Your blood work is showing a false negative, which means there hasn't been enough time for antibodies to develop after the initial exposure. Antibodies fight to suppress foreign bodies in our systems. When there's a delay, the virus is still considered foreign to the body. Most likely, it's your most recent partner," his hands folded onto his lap.

My heart ached a pain I can't even begin to describe. There are no words to describe the emotion that came over me. I immediately thought of the man I'd given my body to for the last seven months. I guess free-love sex really does have its consequences.

"Don't hesitate to give us a call if you have any questions. We know this can be a lot to process," the doctor gave me a print out of my test results and diagnosis. There were so many thoughts running through my mind at once. How was I going to tell him? What if he doesn't know he has it? Will he think I'm responsible for giving it to him? I couldn't be. The doctor said I have a false negative. My body doesn't recognize the virus. I looked over my results which were negative for hsv1 along with the standard STD panel. I left the doctor's office that day in utter dismay. "Thank you," I sniffled on my way out. Sex is idolized so greatly in our society without considering risk factors that come with it. It is unlikely to get tested with casual sex partners prior to a hookup. I did what most would do.

Traffic and pedestrians bombarded me as I stood outside the facility. The sounds of horns beeping drowned out the 90's music playing in the background. I hurried back to work with a lump in my throat and black streaks from mascara running down my face. When work let out, I skipped out on my evening classes. There was no way I was going to be able to make it through the day. I hopped on the L train to the last stop in Brooklyn. My friend suggested that I stay at her house. That way, I wasn't alone while in shock. H E R P E S. The word made me cringe. I felt sick to my stomach in fear of what others would think of me. Saddened by what I thought of myself.

The stigma is fueled by ignorance and lack of proper education and understanding. It forced a shame onto me that I did not deserve to feel. This can be resolved through compassion, communication and empathy towards one another. The stereotype I was up against felt like I was forced to prove my innocence for a crime I did not commit. How could this happen? Why me? Because herpes is like playing Russian roulette. You never know what the outcome will be.

The last time I tried contacting him, I got no response. It wasn't unusual for either of us not to respond when we were unavailable to hookup. However, this was far more urgent than our late night conversations. I wrote to him via text mese stating it was of importance. When I didn't get an immediate response, I asked my friend if I could borrow her phone to make a call. Perhaps an unknown number would provide a reason to pick up.

After just a few rings he answered, "Hello?" "I've been texting you," I said without mentioning my name. He recognized my voice.

"I was just talking about you. I was on the other line when I got your text," he said. "You ignored the last one so I thought you might be doing the same," I took a deep breath gathering my thoughts. "I wasn't ignoring you. I just didn't answer. I was in the middle of something," he paused. This was it. It was now or never. I had to tell him the truth. "What's up?" He asked. "So I got some unfortunate news at the doctor today..." I walked to the front of the house in need of fresh air. There was a nerve wrecking silence before I could finish. "I found out I have herpes."

"Uhm. I'm sorry to hear that," He stuttered.

"Have you been tested for it?" I asked.

"Yeah awhile ago," he said.

"What did they say?" I pushed for more details. "Oh come on! It's my only day off!" He selfishly attempted to dismiss the conversation. "I've had it since I was young. Everyone does," his defense kicked in.

"What? Which one?" I suddenly began to panic.

"One was from kissing my aunt when I was five. And the other...obviously wasn't from my fucking aunt." I froze.

My eyes widened. Till this day, I will never forget the words he spoke. Learning he is positive for both strains not only demonstrated the prevalence of herpes, but also how difficult it is to talk about due to the stigma. What concerned me the most was his inability to put my health before his own agenda.

"You've had it since you were five?" I was astounded. I looked over at my friend. Her face turned to pure horror and lost its color.

"So you gave it to me," I muttered.

"The doctor said I have a false negative. Meaning, it's my most recent partner."

"There are lots of ways you could get it. I was with my girlfriend, ex-girlfriend, for six years and she never got it," He hinted at the possibility I might've contracted hsv from someone else.

"Girls have called me saying they're pregnant. Come to find out there's more to it," he insinuated.

Then it hit me.

He took advantage of me. He took advantage of my body and my trust. He hid his status from me in order to obtain his own benefit. He wasn't my friend. He was the enemy. I hated every part of him.

"I haven't slept with anyone but you recently! Why didn't you tell me?!" I shouted pacing back and forth. "I'm sorry but I'm not obligated to do anything. If the circumstances were different, I'd have told you," He said. "You're not obligated to tell me? Are you serious? It's always about you!" I was confused as to why he would do something so cruel and heartless. "I haven't had an outbreak since

August!" He exclaimed. "That doesn't mean I won't get it! It still transfers. Since you shared something with me, I'm going to share something with you. I broke up with my ex boyfriend and didn't sleep with anyone until you. I've never had this before," I said. Everything was finally starting to make sense. He was hiding from himself.

"What do you need? I'll pay your medical expenses. I can give you dietary options. But read a damn pamphlet before you start coming at me!" He yelled. I remained stunned at the lack of compassion he possessed. His apologies were followed by his crudely insensitive remarks. "Dietary options? I've been calling doctors trying to figure out what was going on with my body. I would rather get information from someone who has it firsthand!" I sobbed. He let out a gentle sigh. "Well, what do you want to know?" He asked. I wanted to send him straight to hell.

"You know what, I don't even feel comfortable talking to you about it anymore. I'm gonna go," I said. "Uh-." I hung up the phone before he could say anything else. My friend gently placed her arm around me caressing my right shoulder. She hugged me as we walked around her neighborhood several times until I was ready to go back inside. "He knew the whole time," I confided in her. "He knew and didn't tell me." My soul was disrupted that night.

He handed me a loaded gun and watched as I pulled the trigger. Unaware of the potential dangers. Flashbacks of his arms wrapped around me as we slept made my skin crawl. His eyes looked deeply into mine before penetration. The inner wound I now processed hurt beyond words can explain.

Because he too was in the dark about my past. The abusive men that came before him. Each of them took a piece of me. I didn't have anymore to give. From the outside looking in, I appeared whole. Locking away years of pain hidden behind my saddened eyes. The next morning, I awoke to a text message from him. You may recognize it from the first chapter. "Destiny, I am truly sorry for everything. I feel terrible. Please let me know how I can help. I want to make this less painful for you. Trust me this is not as bad as it seems."

## Chapter 6

# HEALING

⌒

How deeply regretful it is to have slept with someone like him. He possessed such a cruel mentality towards women. Putting us at risk as he runs and hides from his demons. He is herpes positive. Now, I am too. If I hadn't been so persistent in seeing him, this wouldn't have happened right? Wrong. Self blame never did anyone any good. Each time he lays down with a woman, he is presented with a choice. He actively chooses not to disclose in casual relationships. It took awhile for me to realize in no way was this my fault. It's fair to assume the person we're intimate with maintains a certain level of integrity. On my way to work, I waited at a bus stop in Brooklyn in front of a small bodega. Two middle aged men and an older woman stood nearby. "No one will love you. No one will accept you," my anxiety lied. "This is forever."

My chest tightened as I began gasping for air. "Miss, are you okay?!" They gathered around me. "I can't breathe!" I shouted. Panic attacks.

For me, it went far beyond a herpes diagnosis. This was about deception. Deception and its repercussions. The irreversible damage it can leave upon someone else's life. His dishonesty was accompanied by a terrorizing stigma. One that would haunt me for the rest of my life. I was robbed of my choice. Betrayed by someone who slept with me on numerous occasions for months. Forgiving him was completely out of the question. The concept of moving on with my life and sharing my secret with potential partners didn't come easy. For a while, I avoided every man who took interest in me.

Unresponsive and closed off as they attempt to initiate conversation. Self doubt. I feared rejection would follow a disclosure. Nothing could've been further from the truth. There are exclusive dating sites and confidential support groups. I met herpes positives online who spoke openly about their unique experiences. Discovering I wasn't alone helped me revive. I was able to overcome my initial reaction through time and research. I read tons of online forums and spoke with multiple doctors regarding my diagnosis. The more I educated myself, the easier it became to manage. Each article provided insight on how to come to terms with a positive diagnosis and what options you may have when it comes to sex, treatment, and prevention. There was one in particular that helped me immensely.

The New York State Public Health Laws strictly enforce the disclosure of STDs. It is considered illegal to knowingly, and recklessly transmit an STD. Neglect to inform a sexual partner about your status prior to exposure can result in a misdemeanor or an invasive lawsuit. However, it must be proven that he or she knew of their positive status beforehand. In my case, I was able to pinpoint who my giver was based on my bloodwork and sexual partners within that time frame. Initially, I had zero intentions of suing him or pressing charges. Any added stressors in my life were unwelcomed. I did, however, want him to understand the severity of his careless actions and what he could potentially do to others. Before the court order was in place, I sent him a preview of an article pertaining to New York State Public Health laws and regulations. By no means was it supposed to be taken as a threat. I wanted to prove to him he is in fact obligated to disclose to ALL sexual partners by law. Which includes casualties. "This is bullshit," he said repeatedly asking what I wanted from him. "I didn't expect this from you. I'm hurt," he guilt tripped me. The last thing I expected was for him to give me an STD. One I couldn't rid myself of. There was no holding back my emotions. "Pull yourself together and please talk to me when you do," he wrote.

Generally speaking, no one is under any obligation to disclose their status. We do not have to tell friends, or family members when we have tested positive for an STD. It's confidential. In New York State, it is illegal to knowingly and recklessly transmit an STD if aware of the positive status. Public State Health laws vary from state to state. Myself and countless others are the direct result of what happens when someone chooses to play on words of what obligation means to them. I am elaborating for anyone who may be contemplating whether or not to disclose to their partner. Providing partners with informative consent can protect both persons involved.

Later that week, we spoke over the phone. I sent a message on my way to class demanding we speak in person. "With all the crazy threats you've made? I don't think so," he rejected. I forewarned I would then have to take matters into my own hands. The phone rang within minutes. "What do you want from me?!" He screamed. "I'm not obligated! For someone I'm dating yeah, but not someone I'm just fucking! You're not going to threaten me then have me feeling sorry for you! It's not happening!" His voice heightened through the speaker so loudly I had to pull the phone away from my ear. "I'm not threatening you! I'm hurt! I never did anything for you not to tell me. If you didn't know you had it, this entire situation would be different! You didn't give me a choice!" I screamed back. In the midst of shouting over one another, we became overly emotional. He began confessing his own struggles with being herpes positive.

"I was molested! I didn't have a fucking choice when I got it! So don't talk to me about not having a goddamn choice! If this is the worst thing that's happened to you, you have a lot to learn!" There wasn't a doubt in my mind he had been sexually abused. I knew he was telling the truth. I immediately began sobbing. "I'm sorry that happened to you," I stood aimlessly in front of my school building. While I couldn't begin to comprehend what that must have been like for him growing up, it was not an excuse for careless, erratic behavior. I wouldn't allow him to get away with what he had done to me. Sexual trauma did not deem his behavior acceptable.

"I am sorry. Do you want me to sit here and listen to you tell me how terrible of a person I am? If that's what you need to do to feel better than go ahead! I would never hurt you intentionally. I should have told you but I didn't. So how can we move forward?"

He apologized profusely. "There isn't anything you can do!" I shouted. "That's what happens when you have unprotected sex Princess! You're not innocent!" His brutal words stained my memory. I consented to have unprotected sex under the impression I was safe with him. "Just take the fucking pill!" He yelled once again. If only it were that simple. We wouldn't have been in this situation if he had taken precaution, now would we? With a brief pause, he suggested we should take some time to calm down so we can speak to each other respectfully. It was apparent I needed to cease all communication. But I was conflicted. Holding him legally responsible would mean financial compensation for the future costs of medicine, therapy sessions, maintaining a healthier diet, doctor's visits, emotional distress etc. It was during our last phone call that I came to my final decision.

In order to build evidence against him, I gathered all necessary documents and representation from doctors to support my case. "Why aren't you taking responsibility and helping me?" I asked over the phone. He coughed, "I don't have to take responsibility. I offered my help and you've tried to take full advantage and you're going way too far with it." "How? Can you tell me how I've done that?" I asked. He claimed I was extorting while I hadn't done anything remotely close prior. "Listen man, you're taking this as if you have some death defying illness you suffer from on tragic levels and it's fucking ridiculous!"

He said, "Why didn't you disclose then? If it's not that big of a deal, why didn't you disclose?" I was astounded by his ability to desensitize the issue at hand. "You're treating this like a business matter and it isn't." If I could somehow get him to say he knew his status once more it would strengthen my claim. "I don't know what you're talking about. You've done nothing but been conniving and manipulative," he went on to accuse me of blackmailing him. "Demanding large sums of money, making ludicrous threats of things that are far fucking fetched and far out of the possibility of even truth." He said, I interrupted. "They are truthful though. We know they are," I muttered.

"Okay, fine. Then like I said, if you think that is the case then by all means, I'll see you in court!" He shouted. "Why do that when it's more stressful for the both of us?" I wanted to come to an agreement for a large amount which would contribute to future maintenance of the condition. He declined. "Court isn't going to do shit for you!" He attempted to discourage me.

"As someone with integrity, I didn't think you would be this way," I expressed with deep sadness. "You don't know anything about my level of integrity. I'm very hurt too. All you seem to think about is yourself. You don't give a shit about anyone but yourself!" He said, "I have too many people to support and I'm not going to support you! You wanna ask for something reasonable, I'd be inclined to maybe help you out of the kindness of my heart." He truly sickened me to the pits of my stomach. "The kindness of your heart?! That's what you owe me!" I grew infuriated listening to him speak. "Listen Princess, I have doctor friends, I have lawyer friends, so don't try and take advantage of something you can't do, okay?" He belittled me into thinking I didn't stand a chance against him in court. Defending myself signified the start of something beautiful. Healing. I grew a strength no one can ever take from me. Until this day, I have no regrets about my decision. I stopped writing on many occasions in order to get through the tragic memories he brought me. And this chapter was the most difficult to write by far.

"I need help. The diet is insane." During my transition to hsv2+ (genital herpes positive) it took weeks for my system to develop antibodies. Certain foods triggered my symptoms. In addition to the amount of stress I was under. I was temporarily put on suppressive therapy to relieve me of frequent outbreaks, which added costs. I carefully selected what I ate and began attending therapy regularly. My mental health was severely declining. It was never about the money.

Despite this, I understood I was legally entitled to it. Knowing my rights strengthened my ability to seek justice. No matter how many times he may have disagreed. I've watched society blame the woman for a man's actions far too many times. It's time to put an end to the victim blaming. It's this exact mindset that gives predatory men an escape route. An excuse. "You took advantage of me this entire time," I said. "I didn't take advantage of you. I don't know what you're talking about man. I'll have something for you by the beginning of next week." He proposed a contractual agreement between the two of us. The contract would include a payment which was suitable for him so that he would never have to discuss this with me again.

Three weeks later, he hadn't submitted the contract and I was increasingly running out of patience. He stalled week after week hoping I would eventually leave it alone. It had been a little over a month since my diagnosis and our dilemma went unresolved. We couldn't seem to come to an arrangement on our own. I reached out to him expressing my concerns for other women he would do this to. "I'm going to explore my options and speak to my family because you're not taking this as seriously as you should," I said. He demanded I tell him what I wanted as if I was attempting to extort him. I explained I wanted him to take full responsibility for what he's done.

We agreed on a contract for an amount that would help me financially in the long term. I wanted him to respect his casual sex partners and to stop pretending he didn't know what I was talking about. I questioned how he would feel if someone were to do this to his mother or younger sister. How hurt they would be. How much anger he'd feel towards the person guilty of withholding their positive status.

Predictably, he did not follow through with the contract he proposed. I assume this was a tactic to get me off his back. The following month, I pursued legal action after calling numerous lawyers in Manhattan. A civil suit was then filed against him. Our identities would remain anonymous to the general public. Without my family's involvement and knowing close to nothing about the legal system, I was able to hire a lawyer. While I cannot disclose details of the lawsuit, I can say it worked out in my favor. I won.

After about a year and a half, my case was settled in civil court. The legal process was absolutely dreadful. Suicidal urges became more intense as I fought tremendously in order to remain optimistic. He caused me a great deal of pain and frustration. It was me vs. him in its entirety. I am forever grateful I was given the opportunity for justice to be served. To hold him accountable is wonderfully freeing.

I found my voice to speak up against non disclosure and its devastating impact on someone's life. The lawsuit prevented me from moving forward with my diagnosis for a very long time. It weighed heavily over me like a dark cloud. Everywhere I went, I carried it with me. I am in no way promoting the concept of suing someone for transmission of an STD. I chose to pursue court because my giver has stated he does not believe he is obligated to disclose to all casual sex partners.

In addition, I was able to prove he knew his status prior to my involvement with a sustainable amount of evidence. The lawsuit took a tremendous toll on my mental and emotional health. I experienced the physical symptoms of herpes throughout its entirety due to stress. Fortunately, my outbreaks have lessened over time. I understand no amount of money will ever heal the permanent scars he has given me. Holding him accountable, however, gave me the strength and ability in order to move forward with a life he had disrupted.

His choice not to disclose and lack of human decency developed into a massive loss of trust in people, and severely hindered my sexual confidence until I was able to work through it in therapy. Do not pity me, as I've chosen to open up about what I consider to be a life changing experience. If my story can help one person through the beginning stages of their diagnosis, if I can cause someone to think twice before they make fun of someone with an STI, if I can promote disclosure, then I can honestly say it was all worth it.

I hope to inspire others to become open minded when someone shares their status, and help put an end to the stigma. But I cannot do this alone. I welcome you to be a part of the change. It takes a collective effort for each and every one of us to empathize with one another rather than judge or ridicule someone due to their status. It wasn't until I began disclosing on my own terms that I realized people may not always know how to receive this type of information. It can be tough for both parties involved. But it doesn't have to be. It can be a mature, sex-positive discussion. I can honestly say I've had plenty of successful disclosures. Love after hsv is very much possible. There are options available to secure a healthy, happy relationship with an STD positive. Here are some of the steps which have assisted me during a disclosure:

It is crucial for the person on the receiving end to respect the privacy of the individual sharing their status. It is equally as important to make the other person feel comfortable talking about it. The first step is to enter the conversation as open mindedly as possible. As you would want them to do in return. If the person with a positive status has chosen to discuss this with you, let them. The next step focuses more on discretion. Do not share such intimate information without their permission. Be a good listener by hearing them out entirely; they may answer some of the questions you have. If you would like to learn more about their diagnosis, it could benefit you in the long run. This provides a better understanding as to what they may be experiencing. Take initiative to learn more! It's useful to have conversations about treatment and prevention. The final step is to ask questions. Do not be afraid. They might not want to bombard you with tons of information about statistics, their status, and transmission rates all at once. I ask that we refrain from the usage of the term "clean" when referring to a negative status, as it implies the opposite means dirty.

Let's face it, STDs can be difficult to discuss. We must normalize these conversations to improve sexual education. It can only help change stigma for the better and create a better climate for us all. Get tested. Know your status. Then own it. This should be treated as a standard every time you have a new partner or engage in unprotected sex. The statistics of STDs/STIs are rising due to lack of testing, misinformation regarding transmission and diseases, and fear of disclosure. If needed, please use this book as a guide for anyone struggling with their diagnosis and to inform others on hsv. Herpes does not define me. It's no longer a secret that I am one of thousands who are living successfully as herpes positive. More than half are unknowingly infected with hsv. If you've never experienced an outbreak, it doesn't mean you are in the clear. The most common symptom of an STI is no symptom. Be sure to ask your doctor if you've recently come in contact with an STD to learn more about your status. Herpes is not a consequence or the direct result of poor decision making. Speak your truth. In my last message to him, I remained sincere just as I'd always been. "I'm not angry with you for giving this to me. I'm angry because you did not believe I was worth disclosing to. After all, we were just having fun."

# Chapter 7

# CHANGE

⌒

This is not a cliche love story compiled with romance or a happily ever after. Although my journey has just begun, I am still rebuilding myself and learning throughout my experience. You and I are not an exception. What happened to me can happen to anyone. Each of us have someone close to our hearts living with the virus. They may not speak openly about it or are simply unaware that they have it. Whether it's family members or childhood friends, the majority of the population has a form of herpes. Oral herpes (hsv1) better known as cold sores, is the most popular strand. Other than it's location, it is no different than genital herpes (hsv2). Hsv1 and hsv2 can transmit with or without visible sores or symptoms. I may never know if condoms would have prevented such trauma. What I do know is that I thought I could rely solely on testing.

We risk contracting an STD/STI any time we engage in sexual activity. Hsv can be transmitted through kissing. We risk unknowingly passing the disease onto our partners. No symptom is a symptom. Sleeping with someone who is aware of their status does not increase the risk factor. In fact, becoming knowledgeable about your status makes it a lot easier to keep partners safe. Hsv outbreaks may appear similar to a paper cut or rash. They can be located on the buttocks, inner thighs or within the pubic area. Although it is extremely rare for hsv2 to occur at the mouth, transmission is possible through oral sex. What isn't so rare is the transmission of cold sores on genitals. This is referred to as ghsv1 otherwise known as oral herpes in the genital region. Lack of condom usage or dental dams during oral sex does not necessarily result in fewer risks than penetrative sex. Once someone is infected with hsv in either location, it remains dormant within their nervous system and can spread at any given time. The good news is, outbreaks become slim to none as time goes on after the initial infection and there is a preventative treatment. Talk with your healthcare physician. There are options available in order to keep you and your partner safe. Suppressive therapy is offered as a long term medical prescription used to reduce the number of outbreaks and significantly helps lower transmission rates amongst partners. In simple terms, the medicine works to suppress the virus. Safe sex is still possible! It may also help outbreaks heal faster and reduce possible discomfort.

Now, allow me to put to rest some of the myths you may have heard about herpes. The first being, cold sores are herpes. They are not a fancy exception. This isn't up for debate. It is an STI that is also transmitted through kissing. Neither strain will affect your ability to reproduce. A woman can bear children without further complication. It does not affect fertility in men or women. Life and love goes on with herpes. You can have steaming, hot sex. Hsv positives are not constantly walking around in painful sores. If we were, I'd never leave the house! There is no visible way to tell if someone carries the virus. Symptoms vary from person to person. Outbreaks are commonly mistaken for a rash or ingrown hair. Herpes isn't typically spread through bodily fluids. There would have to be a significant amount of viral load on a shared skin product such as chapstick, during an active outbreak in order for transmission to occur.

The product would then need to be applied directly on the skin after the infected person. Cups, towels, utensils, and clothing are safe to use at discretion. Contraction usually occurs via skin contact! There are safe alternatives used to protect our partners such suppressive therapy which has many benefits as previously mentioned. Not every partner will contract it. It's really a hit or miss considering viral shedding, active outbreaks, condoms, and the use of antivirals. You can sleep with someone hundreds of times and remain negative despite their positive status if precautionary measures are taken such as condoms and suppressive therapy. So how did such a common human virus gain such a poor reputation?

Decades ago, marketing campaigns sought out the opportunity to sell herpes antivirals by instilling fear in all of us. It worked. They projected the horrors of hsv by exaggerating its effects on the human body. The more we feared herpes, the more antivirals, ointment, and other medications they could potentially sell. This means more money for pharmaceutical companies and medical practitioners. There was once a time when herpes wasn't considered as big of a deal as it is today.

Most people were able to heal from outbreaks without medical treatment as their outbreaks were considered minor. Not all outbreaks are painful. At the time, antivirals were considerably expensive and weren't in high demand. To heighten sales, herpes was deemed shameful and boom! This is how the stigma began. Genital herpes was singled out and branded as the scarlet letter, eventually separating from cold sores because of its classification which labeled it an STD. Commercials and advertisements began emphasizing the words "incurable" and "disease" in order to scare the general public to ensure they would sell more products. We believe this concept so greatly, the stigma remains decades later. Women are much more affected by the stigma than men as we are taught to suppress our sexual behaviors.

Herpes is considered one of the most stigmatized conditions till this day. This can make disclosure troublesome. Why should you care about this if you don't have hsv? Because this affects us all by contributing to the spread. I have found within the community, there are far too many of us who do not disclose within casual encounters or in the early stages of relationships due to inconvenience or fear of rejection. Given the significance of hsv, there is a great chance you've already been exposed to hsv. This could be through a kiss on the lips by a relative who has a history of cold sores (hsv1) as a child, or through oral and penetrative sex. Genital skin covers the entire genital area. Inner thighs, anus, and pubic region. Herpes can also occur in monogamous relationships. If one person is unaware that they a carrier, hsv can mistakenly transmit to the other. Rather than judge someone living with the condition, we can become more conscious of its prevalence. Disclosure doesn't have to be a hidden secret reveal. Or a scary conversation before sex. Allow some comfortability into the conversation. Everything is going to be okay. Perhaps, he would have disclosed to me if the stigma didn't exist. While I cannot agree with his decision not to, I can begin to understand why he didn't.

Hsv positives face rejection and humility for a condition which hardly affects our daily lives. You can routinely practice safe sex and test positive. Herpes doesn't necessarily show up immediately. It took me seven months of exposure to contract it. Condoms do not fully protect against hsv and oral contraceptives aren't always consistently used among people who are sexually active. The same strand cannot spread to other parts of your body once antibodies are present. Following initial exposure, the body begins fighting against the virus. However, it is possible to contract both strands in different areas. For example, my giver suffers from cold sores on the mouth in addition to having genital herpes. It is also possible to contract hsv1 and hsv2 in the same region. So what is life with herpes *really* like? I can't speak for every herpes positive out there. I can only speak for myself. For me, it's about adapting to a new sense of self. Self care, self love, and acceptance. Saying to ourselves, "I refuse to punish myself for having a condition which most of the population has. I will not devalue my existence as a human being to make others comfortable. I will continue to love and care for myself." In fact, living with a positive status strengthens our knowledge about sexual health.

Three years ago, I couldn't even begin to imagine that one day my outbreaks would become so insignificant I'd hardly notice. Yet here I am today. I am feeling more confident, openly discussing my status in order to educate others, and taking better care of myself. My outbreaks have slowed down tremendously. I don't remember the last time I had one. Herpes isn't life-threatening. The real setback is how the general public continues to perceive it. My body is completely back to normal and there is nothing gruesome about my lady parts. Most of the time, I forget I have it. It's also common not to experience an outbreak after the initial one. If you are someone who experiences frequent outbreaks like I did when I was newly diagnosed, I want to say that it gets much easier to manage with time. I promise. Staying away from triggers can minimize the number of outbreaks per year. My triggers include stress, catching a cold, chocolate, and nuts. Identify your triggers and take it one day at a time.

Many hsv+ have adopted healthier lifestyles post diagnosis. This is done through exercise to relieve themselves of stressors and strengthen immunity.

Others have improved their diet to combat colds and other viruses. As for me, I now make a conscious effort to better my overall wellness. I practice meditation techniques, treat my outbreaks with natural remedies, and promote healthier lifestyle choices to friends and family. I avoid stressors and listen to my body if it feels run down. When I officially made a year as herpes positive, I anticipated spending the entire day locked in my room grieving the part of me I thought I lost. It took until court was settled to ignite a spark in me again. It wasn't herpes that forced me into a deep depression. It was a betrayal. Hearing him admit he doesn't feel the need to disclose to people he's casually sleeping with. I felt disposable. I was blatantly disrespected. And in that darkness, I found growth. While I am still a work in progress, I have chosen to reclaim my power by shedding light on a stigma that told me no one would ever love me. To silence the voices that said I was partially responsible for what happened to me.

I've spent most of my time in isolation, writing and reflecting. Most importantly we need to see change. Change in the way we think about and discuss STDs. For people such as myself, to be able to share their status without rejection, embarrassment and ridicule. To put an end to the stigma and advocate against non disclosure. If you have tested positive and know your status, I recommend disclosing to all sex partners. Casual hookups, one night stands, and in relationships.

Allow one another to give consent in regards to sexual health. It is never okay to take someone's choice away. Consent to sex does not give to consent to an STD/ STI. If you have a history of cold sores, disclose before the kiss and prior to intimacy. There are antivirals and suppressive therapy medications available to lower transmission rates. Using them along with condoms decreases the chances of transmission. Due to the unpredictable nature of hsv, we can help prevent the spread by getting tested, practicing sex safe and enforcing disclosure. While some may argue STDs/ STIs are inevitable, this is my suggestion to practice safer sex. As previously mentioned, condom use doesn't prevent transmission but it does lower the risk. Hsv is generally passed through the skin. Condoms are designed mainly to protect against fluids. A positive status does not make you unlovable, promiscuous, or dirty. As I previously mentioned, most of us were given a form of herpes as a child. I ask that we keep an open heart when someone chooses to discuss their status. Herpes positives are very capable of having healthy, happy, relationships. It is a personal decision to continue seeing someone following a disclosure.

There is a portion of the herpes community that are self destructive and constantly putting others at risk- repeatedly making the decision not to disclose. I will refer to this group of individuals as serial givers. They are dedicated to putting their needs above all. They are fully aware and well-informed of their status but do not tell partners before sleeping with them. Serial givers contribute greatly to the new cases of herpes as well as other diseases. It isn't done on one occasion or accidentally. It's a repeated decision that is made on numerous occasions at the expense of others. Despite the repercussions, my giver continues to engage in sex without disclosure. And he isn't the only one out there. Serial givers are remotely driven by insecurities, fear, and revenge. They are the people you'd least expect. They are people you trust. If you are someone who has not disclosed your status before sex, it is never too late to do so.

I was surprised to learn that herpes does not discriminate. Hsv positives come in all shapes and sizes, race and ethnic backgrounds. Healthy men and women, celebrities and children are all carriers. It does not reflect our morality whatsoever. I foolishly believed someone who was troubled himself. Someone who hasn't fully accepted himself as hsv positive and what that entails. I trusted the wrong person. And while the stigma has caused him to hide his status from his casual sex partners, I want to ask you, the reader to be a part of the change. Be kind to each other. One of the first herpes jokes I experienced was at work. An old coworker of mine began describing a group of girls she considered trashy from a specific part of the city. "What do they have to act so tough about?" I asked in response to her confrontation with them. "I don't know," she said. "Probably their herpes." My co-workers bursted out in laughter. I froze. Completely stunned by the butt of her joke. Rather than get upset, I chose to educate her. I waited for the others to walk away before pulling her aside. "You know, a lot of people have herpes?" I gently touched her back, "I know someone close to me that has it." I said, "Oh I'm sorry, I was just pissed at those girls," She explained. I didn't mention the closest person to me that has it is me.

Throughout comments on social media and jokes made at bars, stop and think how the person may have contracted the STD/STI. There is a major misconception that the person is sleeping around. What about cheating spouses? A previous relationship where a spouse didn't know? Or when someone with positive status failed to disclose? These scenarios can leave someone with the condition along with the burden of being mocked for it. I have listened to stories of someone who was brutally raped, a virgin who had her first kiss, and an ex-boyfriend who gave it to his girlfriend purposely out of spite. Each scenario has the same outcome. You can be laughing at the joke one day, to become positive yourself.

It has been a long road and at times I wasn't sure if I would make it to see another day. Life isn't easy for anyone. We must keep in mind how deeply our actions can affect someone. You never know what a person is dealing with. If he had been honest with me, a tremendous amount of suffering could have been avoided. But I thank him for showing me what I am capable of and how to be more compassionate towards others. I once asked my therapist if she believed there comes a time when a person can no longer heal from the trauma they've endured throughout their life. They've gone through so much they are no longer able to pick themselves up.

As I sat on the couch, she gave her answer. "I believe you can do everything you want to do. I see those qualities in you. You just have to get past this part first." There is no sense in victim blaming. Focusing on what I could've done differently to prevent the situation or what I should've done will not change it. My choice to sleep with someone I was not in a relationship with did not cause this to happen. I am not the perpetrator. It is extremely important to provide informative consent no matter what the circumstance is.

I hope you walk away with an understanding of the unnecessary embarrassment we force onto one another through ignorance and lack of education. If you are like me and carry an STD, I stand with you. I congratulate you on beating the odds of a vicious and powerful stigma. You are not dirty, do not let anyone tell you otherwise. This is not a consequence of immorality and we are still worth it. We are worth the potential risk of contraction while taking precautionary measures. We are deserving of loving relationships. Genital herpes is one of many venereal diseases. Sexually transmitted diseases come with the territory. Some consider them inevitable. Together, we can tackle the stigma.

Not having a say in my sexual health was absolutely devastating. No one deserves to feel guilty for a communicable illness, curable or not. Don't ever think it can't happen to you. The prevalence of STDs is astounding with hookup culture, inconsistent use of condoms, lack of conversation and misinformation. There is a reluctance to seek and discuss vital information in regards to this topic. It's time we take charge of our sexual health. I ask you, the reader, to refrain from judgement as to how I was given this virus. Rather than focus on the relativity of my message. If we can change how we view STD's, the stigma can no longer exist. The negative impact it serves will no longer thrive. We must change the way each of us view and discuss our sexual health and behaviors. We are all different. Through sharing my journey with each of you, I wish for my words to resonate as this book makes its way into the hands of family members and friends. Lovers and acquaintances. Neighbors and strangers. Spread the message. Spread the word. Spread love.

"The truth will set you free…"

www.ingramcontent.com/pod-product-compliance
Lightning Source LLC
Chambersburg PA
CBHW070810280326
41934CB00012B/3144